Mind Over Weight

Books about Weight Management

Susan Kersley

Published by Susan Kersley, 2024.

MIND OVER WEIGHT

First edition. February 25, 2024.

Copyright © 2024 Susan Kersley.

ISBN: 979-8224092109

Written by Susan Kersley.

Table of Contents

1. Are you overweight?

———

You know you are overweight when your clothes are uncomfortably tight, and you find yourself tugging and adjusting them throughout the day.

Physical activities or everyday tasks that used to be easy now leave you feeling exhausted and out of breath.

People make comments about your weight, which can be hurtful and damage your self-esteem.

You struggle to find clothes that fit well or flatter you and shop in plus-size stores.

You have trouble seeing or reaching certain parts of your body. Tying your shoes or reaching your back when showering is difficult.

Activities such as walking up a flight of stairs or going for a brisk walk are challenging and leave you feeling sore or in pain.

Your doctor expresses concern about your weight and recommends that you lose some weight to reduce your health risks.

You avoid social events or activities because you feel self-conscious about your appearance and worry about how others see you.

Your energy levels are consistently low, and you find yourself relying on unhealthy foods or caffeine to keep you going throughout the day.

You notice changes in your body, such as stretch marks, joint pain, or difficulty sleeping, which may be because of your excess weight.

However, being overweight is not an indicator of your worth as an individual. Whatever your weight, focus on having a healthy lifestyle and loving yourself whatever your weight.

But what to do? You may decide to go on a diet or follow an eating plan to lose some of your excess weight.

There are many confusing plans all persuading you that theirs is the only way to become slim and healthy. But there is no magic formula. Restrictive diets don't work in the long term.

Even if you believe that you eat healthily already, you may be eating too much. You could reduce the size of your portions or decide not to have a second helping. It is said you eat with your eyes, so you can fool yourself by using a smaller dish or piling your plate high with low-calorie, high-bulk foods such as vegetables and salad.

You may try to strike a balance between how healthy a food is against how many calories it has. For example, an avocado is a very healthy choice. It has good fat and plenty of vitamin E - but it has a lot of calories.

In contrast, several spoons of sweet jam have fewer calories than half an avocado. Nutritionally it contains a large quantity of sugar so is not as valuable for your health as an avocado even though it has fewer calories.

Nuts such as walnuts or almonds are good for your health, and contain healthy fat, but are high in calories, although you benefit from having a handful each day.

You could track everything you eat during the day. This enables you to discover ways to eat less. The act of recording what you eat may help you change your eating habits and as a result, lose some of your excess weight.

2. What's stopping you?

There may be several factors that prevent you from losing weight effectively. Here are some you might be facing:

A diet that is high in processed and unhealthy foods can make it difficult to lose weight. It's important to consume a balanced and nutritious diet that includes fruits, vegetables, lean proteins, whole grains, and healthy fats.

Regular exercise is important for weight loss since it helps to burn calories and increase metabolism. If you have a sedentary lifestyle or don't engage in regular physical activity, it can delay your weight loss

Turning to food for comfort to cope with emotions can damage your weight loss efforts. Emotional eating often involves consuming high-calorie, unhealthy foods, which lead to weight gain rather than loss.

A consistent approach to weight loss is essential. If you frequently start and stop diet or exercise plans, it becomes challenging to make progress. Maintaining consistency over time is key for successful weight loss.

Certain medical conditions such as hypothyroidism, polycystic ovary syndrome, or hormonal imbalances can make it harder to lose weight. If you suspect a medical condition is delaying your progress, consult your doctor.

A strong support system can be valuable for weight loss. If you don't have the necessary support from friends, family, or a weight loss community, it can be more challenging to stay motivated and committed to your goals.

Lack of sleep can affect hormones related to hunger and fullness, leading to overeating. Additionally, sleep deprivation can impact energy levels and make it harder to engage in physical activity, delaying weight loss efforts.

Setting unrealistic weight loss goals can set you up for disappointment and frustration. Healthy weight loss is a gradual process, and aiming for steady, sustainable progress is more effective than expecting quick results.

It's essential to develop an approach that suits your lifestyle and needs.

3. Motivation.

———

What would motivate and support you? Some people find motivation from being accountable to a coach, a buddy, or a support group.

One of the principal motivators to lose weight is a desire to improve overall health. Shedding excess weight can reduce the risk of various conditions such as heart disease, diabetes, high blood pressure, and certain cancers. The prospect of enjoying a longer, healthier life can be a significant motivating factor.

Losing weight can lead to increased energy levels and stamina, allowing you to participate in physical activities more easily. This can motivate you to lose weight to achieve a more active and fulfilling lifestyle.

Losing weight can boost your self-confidence and improve your body image. Looking and feeling better about yourself can have a positive impact on various aspects of life, including personal relationships, professional success, and overall mental well-being.

Losing weight can alleviate joint pain, improve flexibility, and allow for increased mobility and ease of movement. The prospect of being able to enjoy physical activities, explore new places, or simply move more comfortably can serve as a strong motivation to shed weight.

Weight loss can lead to improved sleep quality, reducing the likelihood of sleep disorders such as sleep apnoea and snoring. Quality sleep is essential for overall well-being and can improve daytime energy levels, mood, and thinking clearly. The prospect of enjoying better sleep can motivate you to adopt healthy habits and lose weight.

Losing weight can lead to positive social connections and improve relationships with others. Feeling more confident and comfortable in social settings can increase opportunities for positive experiences and create a supportive network that can further encourage you to continue your weight loss.

Each pound or inch lost can be a tangible reminder of the effort and dedication put into reaching your goal. The sense of accomplishment can serve as continued motivation to maintain a healthy weight.

Many people are motivated to lose weight because they want to have a better quality of life as they age. A healthy weight can contribute to significantly reducing the risk of age-related diseases, maintaining independence, and enjoying a higher quality of life in the later years.

4. Letting go of excess weight.

———

If you are sure you want to be slimmer, do you want to know how to do this? You have heard the formula: 'Eat less, eat more healthily and exercise more.' Yet it doesn't always seem to work. You try another diet; the weight initially comes off then is back again when you go back to eating as before.

What can you do?

Think about what food meant to you as a child. It may have been used as a comforter and so has become connected, without you realising it, with love. You need to explore those issues and decide how you can get your need for love and comfort met in other ways than the sugary foods that you've used as a substitute.

Become clear about what you need in your life and then ask for it. Too often you make assumptions about other people and think they can read your mind about what you want and then get very annoyed when they don't do what you hope they would do!

Think beyond the chocolate bar and get your mindset in the right place for letting go of your excess weight, because when you change your mindset, you can change your weight too.

If you are tired of carrying excess weight, both in your body and in your life, then it's time to embrace a healthier, lighter you.

Letting go of excess weight is not just about shedding pounds from your physical body, but also about getting rid of emotional baggage, negative habits, and anything else that no longer serves you. Here are some steps to help you start this life change:

Define what excess weight means to you. Is it a number on the scale, a feeling of heaviness, or something else? Be specific about what you want to let go of, both physically and emotionally.

Focus on nourishing your body with wholesome, nutritious foods and engaging in regular physical activity.

Be more aware of portion sizes and make conscious choices to fuel your body with what it truly needs.

Examine the emotional weight you carry. Identify past traumas, negative beliefs, and toxic relationships that may be dragging you down. Seek therapy or meditation to help release and process these emotions.

Declutter your physical space: Rid yourself of unnecessary belongings, creating a more organised environment. Letting go of material possessions can have a profound impact on your mental and emotional well-being.

Be kind to yourself. Accept that progress may not always be linear, and setbacks are a natural part of personal growth. Treat yourself with patience, love, and understanding.

Surround yourself with supportive friends and family who encourage you. Seek inspiration from like-minded individuals or join communities that support your goals, whether it's fitness, wellness, or personal development.

Develop a positive mindset by reframing negative thoughts, practising gratitude, and visualising your desired outcome. Believe in your ability to let go and embrace a healthier, lighter life.

Letting go of excess weight requires dedication, consistency, and self-reflection. Celebrate every small victory along the way and stay committed to the process.

As you release both physical and emotional weight, you'll discover a newfound freedom and joy within yourself.

5. Become slimmer without a strict diet.

———

You can lose your excess weight when you change your mindset. Your mind is all-powerful and affects the way you eat and the way you look.

Imagine yourself as slim and healthy. See yourself, in your mind's eye, wearing clothes that flatter and fit you perfectly. Hear others telling you how good you look and feel what it would be like to be slimmer and healthier than you are right now.

If you want things to change, you must do something differently. If you continue to eat unhealthy food or fail to exercise, then you will continue to be overweight.

When you are old will you turn around and say, 'OK now I'm ready'? Now I have the time to eat more healthily, do more exercise and find other ways to respond to emotions instead of overeating. Don't delay: the time to make changes is now.

Becoming slimmer doesn't have to involve sticking to a strict diet. While dieting can be effective in achieving weight loss, initially, it doesn't work in the long term. Other approaches can help without following a highly restrictive eating plan.

Here are some tips to help you become slimmer without a strict diet:

Focus on portion control: Instead of cutting out certain foods completely, moderate your portion sizes. Use smaller plates and bowls and become aware of your hunger cues. Listen to your body and eat until you're satisfied.

Incorporate more whole foods: opt for nutrient-dense foods that are both filling and nourishing. Include plenty of fruits, vegetables, lean proteins, whole grains, and healthy fats in your meals. Select whole foods over ultra-processed.

Practice mindful eating by slowing down and savouring each bite. Mindful eating involves paying attention to the taste, texture, and smell of your food, as well as how it makes you feel. This can help prevent overeating and promote a healthier relationship with food.

Stay hydrated by ensuring you're drinking enough water throughout the day. Sometimes, thirst can be mistaken for hunger. Hydration is essential for your body's optimal functioning and can help curb unnecessary snacking.

Get moving by including regular physical activity into your routine. Exercise not only burns calories but also helps boost your metabolism. Find activities you enjoy, such as walking, swimming, dancing, or cycling, and aim for at least 150 minutes of moderate-intensity exercise per week.

Prioritise sleep by aiming for 7-8 hours of quality sleep each night. Sleep deprivation can disrupt your hormones, making it more challenging to maintain a healthy weight. A good night's rest can help regulate your appetite and energy levels.

High stress levels can lead to emotional eating or cravings for unhealthy foods. Find ways to manage stress, such as meditation, deep breathing exercises, yoga, or hobbies you enjoy.

Building healthy habits and making viable lifestyle changes are more effective than extreme dieting. Focus on making small, gradual changes that you can keep to, over time.

Everyone's body is unique, and what works for one person may not work for another. It's important to listen to your body and make choices that feel right for you. If you have any specific health concerns or dietary restrictions, it's always a good idea to consult a healthcare professional or registered dietitian for guidance.

6. Mindset.

———

Having the right mindset to lose weight is essential for achieving your goals and maintaining a healthy lifestyle.

Getting into the right mindset to lose weight requires dedication and perseverance. By adopting a positive and balanced mindset, you set yourself up for long-term success and a healthier and happier life.

Set achievable and realistic weight loss goals for yourself. Instead of focusing on drastic measures, aim for a gradual and sustainable weight loss. This will help you stay motivated and committed in the long run. Weight loss is a gradual process and results may not be immediate. Stay patient and don't get discouraged by any setbacks or plateaus you may encounter.

Reflect on why you want to lose weight. Whether it's to improve your overall health, boost your self-confidence, or increase your energy levels, understanding your motivation will keep you focused on your goals during challenging times.

Instead of viewing weight loss as temporary, think of it as a permanent lifestyle change. This shift in mindset will help you, rather than relying on short-term solutions.

Adopt a positive attitude towards the weight loss process. Instead of criticising yourself for past mistakes or setbacks, focus on your progress and celebrate each milestone. Positive thoughts and self-encouragement will keep you motivated and help you stay on track.

Have a support system of friends, family, or online communities that share similar weight loss goals. Surround yourself with people who understand and support you to provide encouragement and accountability.

Learn about nutrition, exercise, and different weight loss strategies. Educate yourself about healthy eating habits and effective exercise routines to enable you to make informed decisions.

Take care of yourself physically, mentally, and emotionally. Prioritise sleep, manage stress, practice mindfulness, and engage in activities you enjoy. By improving your overall well-being, you'll have the energy and mental clarity needed to stay enthusiastic about your goals.

Trust your intuition and become more aware of messages of physical hunger from your gut.

If you eat too much in response to emotional upsets, then you need to address these. It's a common experience that when people resolve their emotional issues, they lose weight more easily.

Compose three or four positive affirmations to assist your unconscious mind make healthy decisions about food. For example, "I enjoy eating fruit every day," or "I eat when I'm physically hungry."

Write your affirmations on post-it notes and have these in places where you can read them regularly. Also, repeat them to yourself many times every day.

Do something every day that is fun and makes you laugh. This could be reading a few jokes, listening to an audio, or watching a few minutes of a funny video on YouTube.

Practice yoga, Pilates, or Tai Chi regularly. Not only will your physical health improve from the postures you practice, but the concentration needed to do them will increase your mental energy to achieve what you want about losing weight.

Set yourself realistic goals not related to your actual weight, but rather to your improving lifestyle, and your increasing fitness and awareness of healthy nutrition.

Get rid of things in your life which irritate you, whether these are physical such as something which needs repairing, or throwing away, or emotional such as telling somebody what you will or won't be doing any more.

To find the motivation to succeed in your desire to change your weight and become healthier you need to have the right mindset. Are you often pessimistic? Are you open to new possibilities or stuck in a fixed mindset? Understanding where you currently stand will help you recognise areas that need improvement.

Changing your mindset takes time and effort. It requires consistent practice and a commitment to developing new habits. Be patient with yourself and celebrate small victories along the way. Lasting change is a gradual process.

Changing your mindset can have an overwhelming effect on your overall well-being and success. Once you have the right mindset about what to eat and what to stop eating, then you can achieve the healthy weight you want.

What's the very first thing to do? Think of how you would like to be when you are at your ideal weight. Take a few minutes each day to sit quietly and imagine how you would like to look. The more you think about this image the more likely it will happen.

Become familiar with what foods are important to eat more, and those which you should limit to some extent.

- Trust yourself to make the right choices.
- Learn about food and what your body needs.

- Be adventurous and try different foods.
- Have a variety of healthy plant-based foods.
- Increase plant-based fibre: nuts, seeds, and beans.
- Fill up on fruit, and vegetables.
- Stop eating ultra-processed food.

Become aware of your natural messages of physical hunger.

Getting into the right mindset is crucial for achieving success and overcoming challenges. It involves cultivating a positive and focused attitude that enables you to approach tasks and obstacles with determination and resilience.

Identify what you want to achieve. Having a specific goal in mind gives you a sense of purpose and direction. Goal setting is an essential part of changing your mindset. Set realistic goals that align with your desires and values. Break them down into smaller, achievable steps, and celebrate your progress along the way. This practice not only helps you stay motivated but also reinforces a positive mindset.

Imagine achieving your goal. Picture the steps you need to take and the positive outcome you will experience. This technique helps create a positive mindset.

Instead of dwelling on past mistakes or worrying about future challenges, concentrate on the present moment. By being fully present, you can give your best effort and make progress towards your goal.

Focus on the positive aspects of any situation. Look for opportunities instead of obstacles. Surround yourself with positive people, uplifting environments, and inspiring thoughts.

Develop a habit of expressing appreciation for the things you have and the progress you make. Gratitude shifts your mindset from a scarcity mentality to an abundance mentality, cultivating a positive outlook.

Cultivating an attitude of gratitude can have a significant impact on your mindset. Start by acknowledging things you are grateful for each day. This practice shifts your focus from what's wrong to what's right and helps you appreciate the positive aspects of your life.

When negative thoughts arise, challenge them with positive affirmations. Replace thoughts like "I can't do this" with "I am capable of overcoming challenges and achieving my goals."

Read books, watch videos, or listen to podcasts that inspire and motivate you. Learning from the experiences of others can encourage you and provide insights into how to approach your challenges.

Maintaining a healthy lifestyle can greatly impact your mindset. Eat nutritious food, exercise regularly, and get enough sleep. When your body feels good, your mind is more likely to be in the right state for success.

Instead of fearing failure, see it as an opportunity to learn and grow. Consider what went wrong, take lessons from the experience, and use them to improve and try again.

Build a network of supportive individuals who believe in you and your goals. Their encouragement and feedback can help you stay motivated and focused.

Getting into the right mindset is an ongoing process. Practice these steps consistently, and gradually, you will find yourself developing a positive, motivated, and determined mindset that can propel you towards success.

When you change your self-talk about what's going on you really can change the way you feel about it.

Limiting beliefs are thoughts that hold you back and prevent you from reaching your full potential. Identify the beliefs that are holding you back and challenge them. Ask yourself if they are rational or if they are based on fear or past experiences.

Start paying attention to your thoughts and challenge any negative or self-defeating ones. When a negative thought arises, replace it with a positive or more realistic one. For example, if you catch yourself thinking, "I'll never be able to achieve this," reframe it to, "I may face challenges, but if I work hard and stay focused, I can achieve my goals."

Choose to spend time with people who have a positive mindset and encourage personal growth. Avoid individuals who consistently bring negativity or doubt into your life. Surrounding yourself with positivity can have a profound impact on your own mindset.

Adopt a growth mindset, which means viewing challenges and failures as opportunities for learning and growth rather than as roadblocks.

Practice mindfulness and self-awareness by being mindful and self-aware, you can catch negative thoughts and emotions early on and choose to redirect your focus. Engage in activities that promote mindfulness, such as meditation, journaling, or spending time in nature.

Seek personal development with activities that promote personal growth. Read books, attend seminars, take courses, or work with a mentor or coach who can help you gain new perspectives and challenge your current mindset.

An important skill to have when you want to lose weight is being assertive. This means:

- Saying 'no' when you mean 'no'
- Not letting others persuade you to do things you don't want

to do.

- Not letting others decide what you will eat.
- Recognising what you want.
- Not avoiding things because you don't want to upset someone.
- Being selfish about looking after yourself.

Changing your mindset can be a powerful tool in transforming your life and achieving your goals. By shifting the way you think and perceive situations, you can develop a more positive outlook and create opportunities for growth and success.

7. Change mindset to change weight.

———

Let go of assumptions about how to lose weight and think of different ways to succeed. When you are stuck, use your creativity to challenge your beliefs about diet and weight loss. You could challenge your assumptions by asking yourself:

- On what evidence do I think so and so?
- If I no longer dieted, what might be the worst thing that could happen?
- What might be the best thing that could happen?
- What stops me being the weight I'd like to be?

Then try visualisation or daydreaming. As you close your eyes and relax your body from head to feet, let your mind drift as you imagine yourself as the person you'd like to be. Notice how you look, how you behave, your posture and your expression. Your challenge is to bring some of that into your life now.

For example, wear the sort of clothes the 'ideal you' wears. If the 'ideal you' were taking part in an activity you would like to do 'when you've lost some weight' then start now, whatever your weight.

What are you really frightened of? Is that true, or is it your assumption? What do you need to succeed? For example, if you need more confidence, then think of a time when you felt really, confident. Recall how you felt and when the feeling is very strong then 'anchor' it by pressing your index finger and thumb together. Repeat this several times so that you condition yourself to respond with confidence whenever you press your finger and thumb together.

Weight gain or loss is not just about the physical aspect, but also about our thoughts, beliefs, and behaviours. By changing your mindset, you can develop healthier habits, adopt a positive outlook, and ultimately achieve your weight goals.

Negative thoughts can sabotage your weight loss efforts. Become aware of your inner critic and start challenging those negative patterns. Remind yourself of your capabilities, inner strength, and worthiness of a healthier lifestyle.

Don't set yourself up for failure by aiming for unrealistic weight loss targets. Instead, set small, achievable goals that are specific, measurable, attainable, relevant, and time-bound (SMART). Celebrate each milestone, no matter how small, and use it as motivation to keep going.

Weight loss comes with ups and downs. Instead of beating yourself up over a setback or slip-up, treat yourself with kindness, understanding, and forgiveness. Remember that mistakes happen, and what matters is how you respond and get back on track.

Many people view exercise as a chore or punishment. Change your .by reframing exercise to nourish and care for your body. Find physical activities that you genuinely enjoy, whether it's dancing, hiking, or yoga. Exercise should be a source of joy and self-care rather than just a means to burn calories.

Weight loss is not just about diet and exercise but also about overall well-being. Adopt a holistic approach by focusing on nourishing your body with nutritious food, getting enough quality sleep, managing stress, and practising self-care. A healthy mind and body go together.

Do you live most of the time in your head? You dash about analysing, discussing, deciding, and thinking. You grab a bar of chocolate here or a bag of crisps there; you don't stop for lunch unless it's a big business lunch. This means you either don't have enough or you overeat and have too many unhealthy snacks or meals.

It doesn't have to be that way. You can change your mind and stop being overweight once and for all.

What do you have to do to achieve the weight you always wanted and be healthy too?

Weight loss is easy when you do it by connecting with your body. Your body can communicate in ways that your head may not. It can be very helpful or useful to notice what happens to your body. What is your overweight body saying to you?

Are you tense, relaxed, excited, or sad? These are emotions you may not have thought come from your body, more than from your head. When you feel sad, for example, your body posture will change. So, it's important to connect to these changes.

Do you eat to push those feelings away? Wouldn't it be wonderful to find a way to address your mind and so help your body lose some of its excess weight?

It's important to discover not only what your body is desperate for, but also which part of your body is metaphorically crying.

Where are the areas of tension in your body, especially when you are overwhelmed with a desire to eat too much? If you can become aware of the tension, then ask yourself what happened just before you felt that tension.

As you notice these things you can become more aware of the way your mind and body are interconnected, and how your body is telling you something.

When you connect with your body you begin to listen to those voices. If you can't hear anything yet then take a few minutes to sit quietly with your eyes closed and scan through your body from head to feet, noticing as you go if any area feels tense.

8. Take a moment to pause.

———

C lose your eyes and bring your attention inward. Take a deep breath in and slowly exhale, allowing any tension or stress to melt away.

Begin by scanning your body from head to toe, noticing any areas of tightness or discomfort. Without judgment or trying to change anything, simply observe how your body feels in this present moment.

Now, gradually move your focus to your breath. Feel the gentle rise and fall of your chest, the sensation of the air entering and leaving your lungs. Allow your breath to anchor you in the present, as it is always happening in the here and now.

Bring your attention to your hands. Notice the warmth or coolness, the softness or firmness of your palms and fingers. Wiggle your fingers and be fully present with the sensation of movement. As you connect with your hands, you're acknowledging the incredible capacity of touch and dexterity they possess.

Transfer your attention up to your arms and shoulders. Feel the weight and strength in your upper limbs. Take a moment to appreciate all the actions they allow you to perform - hugging, reaching, creating, and more.

Shift your attention now to your legs and feet. Become aware of the support they provide you as you stand and move through life. Notice the feeling of your feet connecting with the ground beneath you, grounding you in the present moment. Feel the muscles in your legs, acknowledging their power and flexibility.

Now, expand your awareness to your entire body. Feel the energy flowing through you, the aliveness in every cell. Appreciate the remarkable vessel that is your body, enabling you to experience the world and all its wonders.

As you take one more deep breath, gently return your attention to the surroundings, opening your eyes. Carry this newfound connection to your body with you throughout your day, reminding yourself to be present and grateful for all that your body allows you to do and experience.

9. Weight loss basics.

———

L osing weight can be challenging for many people. However, with the right approach, it is possible to achieve your weight loss goals healthily and sustainably.

The first step is to set realistic and achievable goals. Be patient, and allow yourself enough time to make gradual progress. Aim for a loss of 1-2 pounds per week to ensure long-lasting results.

Focus on eating a balanced diet that includes plenty of fruits, vegetables, whole grains, lean proteins, and healthy fats. Avoid ultra-processed and sugary foods, as they can hinder your weight loss progress.

Pay attention to your hunger and fullness cues. Eat slowly and mindfully, savouring each bite. This approach allows you to enjoy your meals and enables your body to register fullness more effectively, preventing overeating.

Regular physical activity is essential for weight loss and overall well-being. Find activities you enjoy and make them a part of your routine. Aim for at least 150 minutes of moderate-intensity or 75 minutes of vigorous-intensity activity each week, and strength training exercises for muscle development.

Stress and emotions can trigger unhealthy eating habits. Find alternative ways to manage stress, such as meditation, yoga, or engaging in hobbies you enjoy. If you find yourself reaching for food due to emotional reasons, practice mindful eating and seek support.

Drinking enough water throughout the day is essential for optimal digestion, metabolism, and overall health. It can help control hunger pangs and prevent overeating. Aim for at least 8 glasses of water per day and increase your intake during exercise or hot weather.

Adequate sleep is vital for weight loss as it affects hormones that regulate appetite and metabolism. Aim for 7-9 hours of quality sleep each night to support your weight loss efforts. Establish a regular sleep schedule and create a relaxing evening routine to improve sleep quality.

Keep a record of your food intake, exercise routine, and overall progress. This will help you identify patterns, adjust, and stay motivated throughout your losing weight. Utilise weight loss apps, fitness trackers, or a simple journal to document your achievements.

Weight loss doesn't have to be a disheartening task. By following these practical tips and applying them to your daily routine, you can make your weight loss more manageable and successful.

Stay committed, patient, and kind to yourself throughout the process. Focus on your long-term health and well-being and celebrate every milestone along the way.

10. Has a problem taken over your life?

———

D o you wonder whether you should do this or do that and although you try to talk to your nearest and dearest or your colleagues all that happens is that they either tell you what they would do (which doesn't appeal to you at all) or encourage you to get on with your life and stop worrying.

Either way, you still don't know what to do and your health is beginning to suffer as a result. You lie awake each night worrying and the dark shadows under your eyes are there for all to see.

You aren't eating properly, filling up on sugary snacks as a way of comfort eating or have lost your appetite for healthy food. Your weight has started to increase dramatically.

What can you do? You could find someone to support you such as a coach or a counsellor.

You will be able to talk to that person and get the support you need from someone who is there to listen to your ideas and who will comment in a way which will help you come to your way forward.

Use the writing technique of 'flow of consciousness.' Acquire a notebook to be your journal and write in it every day. Write until you have covered several pages in writing with whatever comes into your mind. Keep your pen on the paper and don't edit what you write. Each day when you have finished writing put a book-mark in the journal so the next day you can carry on where you left off. Date your entries but don't re-read, just write.

At first, you use the exercise to dump your frustration and other emotions about the challenge you must deal with and then, after a while, you begin to write about possibilities and actions you might take and clarify your thoughts to move forward.

Writing will improve not only your emotional but also your physical health so you can move away from your worries and take the appropriate actions to live the life you want.

If a problem takes over your life and you find yourself consumed by an issue that it affects your daily routine, relationships, and overall well-being, then you are not alone. Many people are trapped in a vicious cycle, where a problem or challenge becomes overwhelming and starts to control every aspect of their life.

Whether it is a health concern, addiction, financial struggles, relationship difficulties, or any other problem, it can feel like an insurmountable obstacle. It may seem like there is no escape, and all your energy and focus are redirected towards dealing with this issue.

The repercussions of having such a problem can be devastating. Your mental and emotional health might suffer as you worry about the situation. You may experience a loss of concentration and performance in other areas of your life, such as work or school. Your relationships may deteriorate as you become consumed by the problem, distancing yourself from loved ones who may offer support.

Living with a problem that has taken over your life can affect your ability to cope with other challenges. It prevents you from fully enjoying life and pursuing your goals.

However, you have the power to regain control and break free from this cycle. Acknowledging the problem and seeking help is the first step towards finding a solution. Reach out to friends, family, or professionals who can offer guidance and assistance.

Engaging in activities such as exercise, relaxation techniques, or hobbies can provide a sense of relief and perspective. Focusing on other aspects of your life that bring you fulfilment can help reduce the overwhelming impact of the problem.

With determination, support, and proper resources, you can regain control, find balance, and move towards a happier and healthier life.

11. Less stress.

———

I f you eat too much when you are already stressed, then finding ways to deal with this will have a beneficial effect and change your eating habits too.

Losing weight itself can be challenging and stressful. However, it's important to find ways to make the process more enjoyable and less overwhelming. By using certain strategies and mindset shifts you can reduce stress levels and increase your chances of success.

Rather than thinking about what you can't have, shift your mindset towards nourishing your body with wholesome foods. Consume a variety of nutrient-dense foods, such as fruits, vegetables, lean proteins, and whole grains that will fuel your body and provide the necessary energy for weight loss.

Find ways to move your body that you genuinely enjoy. Whether it's dancing, swimming, walking, or playing a sport, taking part in activities that you find fun will help you reduce stress. Regular exercise is a proven stress reliever. Activities like brisk walking, swimming, or dancing can help reduce stress levels and promote weight loss. Choose activities that you enjoy, as your motivation to exercise regularly will increase.

Instead of focusing on the end goal, celebrate your small milestones along the way. Recognise and appreciate even the smallest achievements you make, whether it's choosing a healthier option at a meal or completing a challenging workout. This positive reinforcement will help you stay motivated and reduce stress. It's essential to find what works best for you.

Some people eat too much in response to anger, sadness, or frustration. Identify how you feel. Is there a particular person involved when you get those feelings? Where are you when it happens? Is it about your self-esteem or your beliefs about who you are and what you are capable of?

Become more aware of what is happening to you, your mind and your body and the way you respond. If you change one of these then other changes will happen too. For example, if you notice you feel like eating too much after an argument with your partner then decide you won't get into that conversation again. Notice how it starts and be ready with a strategy to change your response. This could be that you say something different, or you physically leave the room. When you feel tension building, don't rush to eat something. Instead, take some slow breaths in and out. As you breathe in say to yourself, 'I'm breathing in calmness and relaxation,' and as you breathe out, 'I'm breathing out tension and anger,' (or whatever negative emotion you feel at the time).

Stress can significantly impact your body's ability to lose weight, as it triggers hormonal imbalances and affects your eating patterns. By adopting strategies to reduce stress, you create a more favourable environment for weight loss.

Engaging in activities such as yoga, meditation, or deep breathing exercises encourages relaxation, reduces anxiety, and calms your mind. Regular practice lowers stress levels and improves your ability to manage your emotions effectively.

Adequate sleep is crucial for weight loss as it affects hormones involved in appetite control. Lack of sleep increases levels of the hunger hormone, ghrelin and decreases levels of the satiety hormone, leptin, leading to overeating.

Take time for yourself and take part in activities that bring you joy and relaxation. Whether it's reading a book, taking a warm bath, listening to music, or spending time in nature, find activities that help you unwind and recharge.

Be aware of your eating habits and pay attention to the sensations of hunger and fullness. When you eat mindfully, focus on the taste, texture, and smell of your food, which can help you recognise when you have eaten sufficiently and prevent overeating.

Ensure your diet includes essential nutrients, vitamins, and minerals to support your body's functions. Avoid relying on ultra-processed or sugary foods as these can exacerbate stress and hinder weight loss progress. Instead, choose whole, unprocessed foods like fruits, vegetables, lean proteins, and whole grains.

Avoid putting excessive pressure on yourself to lose weight quickly. This can lead to more stress and potential setbacks. Instead, set realistic and achievable goals, focus on adopting healthy habits, and celebrate every small success along the way.

Weight loss involves taking care of not only your physical health but also your mental and emotional well-being. By implementing these strategies to reduce stress, you can create a more balanced lifestyle that supports your weight loss goals.

12. What I've learned.

———

O ver many years of trying to reach my 'ideal weight', I've learned some things about weight loss.

I have learned it is not about:

Following a strict formula: There are many so-called "new diets" that rely on either including or excluding, certain foods, eating at certain times of day or barring some food groups entirely. Although, initially weight is lost, the rules and restrictions are not viable in the long term, so the weight returns since it is almost impossible to keep to the rules in the long term.

Counting calories or points is difficult. It is a challenge to consistently keep a record of precisely what you eat. It is doable for a while to weigh and measure food, yet you must live your life, as well as trying to lose weight. After a while, you can no longer count calories, exclude certain food groups from your diet or eat meals as prescribed so you give up completely and feel you have failed.

Being healthy is not only about weight change: it's about enjoying life. That means being able to join social events, eat with friends, and go to parties. When you force rigid rules onto yourself your body reacts by craving what you are trying to stop or going into starvation mode which means that you put on weight more readily even though your intake has gone down.

Instead, you could: Become aware of healthy foods so what you eat is good for your body and your general health and satisfies your genuine physical hunger.

Become more aware of when you turn to food for emotional reasons and learn how to deal with those feelings in other ways apart from eating.

Bring more exercise into your daily routine, without being fanatical, because exercise keeps your body working efficiently. The more you introduce regular exercise the more likely you are to feel better about yourself and to eat in response to the physiological needs of your body rather than to its emotional needs.

Accept that there are days when you eat more and days when you eat less.

Be more relaxed about eating, exercise and weight change and trust the process that happens quite naturally when you change your mindset about your weight.

Let go of old messages about food. Your beliefs about food may have come from your parents when you were a child but as an adult, you need to let go of opinions such as:

- I should eat everything on my plate.
- Don't waste food.
- If you eat it all you can have a pudding.
- Eat what I cooked for you.

Rephrase these by adding 'if I choose.' Instead of 'I should'.

For example:

- I clear my plate if I choose.
- I waste food if I choose to do so.
- I have a pudding if I choose.
- I eat what you cook if I choose.

When it comes to losing weight, I now know that it is not just about following a specific diet or hitting the gym every day. It is a lifestyle change that involves various aspects of your life.

Here are a few key lessons:

It starts with the right mindset. Losing weight requires commitment, discipline, and patience. It is important to believe in yourself and set realistic goals. Being mentally prepared and determined makes weight loss much easier.

A balanced and nutritious diet plays a critical role in losing weight. I have learned that it is crucial to feed my body with wholesome foods that are rich in vitamins, minerals, and fibre. Opting for lean proteins, fruits, vegetables, and whole grains while limiting ultra-processed foods and sugary snacks has helped me make progress.

Portion control is part of weight loss. Learning to listen to my body's hunger and fullness cues has been helpful. Instead of mindlessly eating, I have started to savour every bite, practising mindful eating. This way, I become more aware of when I am satisfied and avoid overeating.

Regular physical activity is essential for weight loss. From cardiovascular exercises like running, swimming, or cycling to strength training and yoga, finding a form of exercise that I enjoy has made it easier to stay committed. Exercise not only helps burn calories but also boosts overall health and well-being.

I learned that consistency is essential for achieving and maintaining weight loss. Establishing healthy habits and sticking to them is crucial. From eating well-balanced meals to exercising, these are choices that help to create positive lifestyle changes.

Losing weight is not an overnight process. It takes time, effort, and dedication. It is important to be patient with the progress and not be too hard on oneself. Self-care is vital during weight loss to maintain a healthy mindset and stay motivated.

Support can make a huge difference to your weight loss. Having people who understand and motivate you can help overcome obstacles and keep you accountable.

In conclusion, losing weight goes beyond just numbers on a scale. It requires a shift in mindset, healthy eating choices, regular physical activity, consistency, patience, and self-care. I have learned that losing weight becomes not just a goal but long-term lifestyle changes that result in a healthier and happier life.

13. Your environment.

———

I t has been said that your environment reflects your subconscious. When inanimate objects start to break down and need repairing take a moment to reflect what connection there might be between your outer and inner world.

Has your washing machine stopped working when you are stressed about having visitors and you need to wash a load of extra sheets and bed linen? It's remarkable how often you find connections and how clearing clutter has so much benefit.

Unlikely as it might seem, when you finally do the tasks that you've been avoiding for ages, your stress, and your desire to overeat will both decrease.

Clutter affects you. Here is a tip to help you to feel better about yourself, eat less and lose weight. It's a simple thing to do, so simple that you may not believe until you try what a great effect it will have on you and your life. If you tend to overeat when feeling stressed, then this will lead to less stress and so you will no longer need to overeat.

What you must do is to clear your clutter. Yes, when you become tidier and throw away what you no longer need or want, the result will be less stress and you can say goodbye to overeating too.

Look around your home. Start with the room you are in right now and ask yourself what you could do to make it look tidier and less cluttered.

If you have surfaces covered in old newspapers or letters, unwashed cups or plates, packaging or bits and pieces, start right now to sort these out.

You can do this section by section such as one surface at a time or one cupboard then a drawer as you gradually sort out your belongings and re-arrange them in a more orderly way.

Have boxes into which you can put things for recycling or charity shops.

Store the things you want to keep in a more organised way, so you know where to find them. You may discover you have something you've been looking for that you'd forgotten where you'd put it.

Clear out unhealthy foods from your refrigerator and cupboards and keep the work surfaces uncluttered. You are more likely to prepare and eat healthy meals when you have a clear kitchen filled with good quality food than when you live in a mess.

The bonus is that living in a clear and uncluttered home will enable you to feel relaxed, happier, and less stressed and so eliminates the need to go to the food cupboard to relieve tension.

Your environment reflects your thoughts, feelings, and mindset. Just as your inner self can shape and influence your external environment, your external environment can also shape and influence you internally.

Consider a cluttered and disorganised space. It may reflect a chaotic and cluttered mind. The state of your physical environment affects your mental and emotional well-being. When you are surrounded by mess and chaos, it can create feelings of overwhelm and stress. In contrast, a clean and organised space can provide a sense of peace and calmness.

The type of environment you choose to surround yourself with can also reveal aspects of your personality and interests. Your home decorations, the colours you choose, the books on your shelves, and the artwork you display can all reflect your preferences, values, and passions. It can give people a glimpse into your identity and what matters most to you.

More than your physical surroundings, the people you choose to spend time with, also influence you. Your social environment can impact your thoughts, beliefs, and behaviours. Surrounding yourself with positive and supportive individuals can uplift your mood and encourage personal growth. Conversely, toxic, or negative relationships can drag you down and hinder your progress.

The natural environment you immerse yourself in can have a profound effect on your well-being. Being in nature, such as going for a walk in a park or hiking up a mountain, can provide a sense of tranquillity and connection. It can help you feel grounded and centred, allowing you to tap into your subconscious mind.

In addition, how you interact with your environment can speak volumes about who you are. Do you take care of your surroundings? Do you respect and appreciate nature? Do you leave places better than you found them? These actions can reflect your values and level of consideration for others.

Taking care of your environment can act as a reminder to take care of yourself and encourage a positive mindset.

14. Keep on top of clutter.

———

C lutter has a habit of re-forming frequently so if you have a clear-out session from time to time, you may find that after a few weeks or months, the problem is as bad as before. It's important to develop a regular clutter-clearing habit.

Any routine may be difficult to implement at first. However, a new habit will eventually become something that you do without thinking. Being tidy and clearing, donating, or selling things you no longer need will have very positive benefits for you. You become:

- Less stressed.
- Happier in a clutter-free environment.
- More focussed in your thinking.
- Able to resist eating too much.
- Able to prepare healthy and tasty meals.
- More organised.
- More able to complete tasks.

Keeping on top of clutter can be a constant struggle for many people. However, with some simple strategies and habits, you can maintain a clutter-free environment and promote a sense of calm and focus in your daily life.

Make decluttering a regular part of your routine. Set aside a specific time each week or month to go through your belongings and get rid of items you no longer need or use. This will prevent clutter from accumulating over time.

Assign specific places for different items in your home or workspace. This will make it easier to put things away and find them when needed. Use storage bins, shelves, or drawers to keep everything organised and neatly stored.

Whenever you bring in a new item, commit to getting rid of something else. This rule helps prevent the accumulation of unnecessary items and keeps your space from becoming overwhelmed with things you don't use.

Dedicate just five minutes each day to tidying a specific area. Whether it's your kitchen counter, desk, or living room, spending a few minutes to put things away will prevent clutter from piling up.

Use filing cabinets or digital folders for important documents and papers. Have different categories such as bills, receipts, medical records, etc. This will prevent paperwork from cluttering your desk or countertops.

Regularly clean your living space to prevent dirt and clutter from accumulating. Set aside specific days or times for different cleaning tasks, such as vacuuming, dusting, or washing dishes.

Go through your belongings and get rid of duplicates or similar items you don't need. Having fewer duplicates will save space and make it easier to find and maintain what you have.

Instead of throwing away items you no longer need, consider donating them to charity or selling them online. This not only helps declutter your space but also benefits others who may find value in these items.

When you pick up an item, don't put it down in a different spot. Immediately decide where it belongs and put it back in its designated place. This prevents unnecessary clutter build-up.

Before buying something new, ask yourself if you need it and if you have space for it. Being mindful of your purchases will prevent unnecessary clutter from entering your home or workspace. Keeping on top of clutter is an ongoing process, so be patient with yourself. By implementing these strategies and making them a part of your routine, you'll be able to maintain a clutter-free environment and enjoy a more organised living space.

Clearing clutter not only helps you create a more organised and peaceful living environment but can also aid in your weight loss journey. Here's how clearing clutter can help you shed those extra pounds:

A cluttered living space can often cause mental distractions and decrease focus. By clearing clutter, you create an environment that encourages concentration and mindfulness. This focus and mental clarity can help you stay committed to your weight loss goals and make more conscious choices about your eating habits.

Cluttered surroundings can lead to increased stress levels, which can trigger emotional eating. Stress and clutter both create a sense of overwhelm and can cause you to seek comfort in unhealthy food choices. Clearing clutter can decrease stress, giving you a better chance of making healthier choices.

Clearing clutter requires physical activity, whether it's organising, cleaning, or moving things around. Engaging in these activities can increase your daily movement and contribute to calorie burning. You'll be surprised how much you can work up a sweat while decluttering your home.

Having a clean, well-organised kitchen encourages you to opt for nutritious foods and makes it easier to find ingredients for healthy meals. On the other hand, a cluttered kitchen may make it difficult to find healthy options, leading to mindless snacking or reliance on processed foods.

A cluttered bedroom can interfere with your sleep quality. Poor sleep affects your hormone balance and can lead to weight gain or difficulty losing weight. By clearing the clutter from your bedroom, you create a peaceful and relaxing environment, allowing for better sleep hygiene and improved weight management.

Clearing clutter is not just about physical objects; it also involves letting go of emotional baggage and negative associations. Releasing these emotional attachments promotes a positive mindset for your weight loss. When you are emotionally lighter, you are more likely to make healthier choices for your body and mind.

Ultimately, clearing clutter is about creating a supportive living environment that supports your weight loss goals.

By removing physical and emotional clutter, you create the space and mindset necessary to focus on your health and well-being.

15. The body-mind connection.

―――――

There are phrases we use commonly such as 'butterflies in my stomach' 'not flexible enough' 'heartache' that are used to express feelings in parts of the body.

Your body gives useful information. You need to listen to your 'inner voice', that gives you a 'gut feeling' about something. Have you ever chosen to ignore it, and then experience consequences which could have been avoided if you had listened?

Have you noticed how sometimes, after a discussion about the pros and cons of making this decision or that decision, you end up making one that 'feels right'?

Instead of dismissing the connection between body and mind, it's vital to not only acknowledge it but also to listen to what it has to say to you. The next time you notice some discomfort in your body take a few moments to sit quietly, concentrate on that part and ask what it is telling you. You may be surprised at the insights this gives you.

Similarly, when you have a strong desire to overeat unhealthy food be more alert to clues within yourself that may indicate the reason for this.

You may find that overeating happens when you feel depressed, anxious, or sad. If you can recognise these connections then you will be in a better position to deal with, or accept, the underlying cause.

The body-mind connection is the interrelationship between your body and your emotional state. It has been a topic of debate in psychology, medicine, and philosophy, the idea is growing that such a connection does indeed exist.

Numerous studies have shown the influence of psychological and emotional states on physical health. For example, stress and anxiety have been linked to a range of physical conditions, including cardiovascular diseases, gastrointestinal disorders, and weakened immune function. The release of stress hormones, such as cortisol, can have detrimental effects on the body over time. Conversely, positive emotions like happiness and contentment have been associated with better overall health and well-being.

On the other hand, your physical state can impact emotional well-being. Hormones, neurotransmitters, and other biochemical substances in the body play a crucial role in regulating mood and cognitive function. Imbalances in these chemicals can lead to mental health disorders, such as depression or anxiety.

Various forms of mind-body practices, like yoga, tai chi, and meditation, have been used to strengthen the body-mind connection. These involve physical movements or postures combined with mental focus and relaxation techniques. Research has indicated that these practices can have positive effects on both physical and mental health. For instance, mindfulness meditation has been shown to reduce stress, improve cognitive function, and even alter the structure and function of the brain.

Advances in neuroimaging technologies, such as magnetic resonance imaging (fMRI), have provided evidence of the body-mind connection. Studies utilising fMRI have demonstrated how specific mental states or emotional responses can affect different regions of the brain. Changes in brain activity and connectivity have been observed in response to stress, meditation, and even placebos.

The body-mind connection is complex. It comprises the relationship between physical health and mental well-being. The evidence supporting this connection continues to grow, and its implications for healthcare and overall wellness cannot be overlooked. Recognising and nurturing this connection can potentially lead to a more all-inclusive approach to health, where both the body and mind are engaged in promoting overall well-being.

16. Nurturing body, mind, and spirit.

―――

When you decide it's time to look after your body by eating more healthily, you will notice good effects on your mind and spirit too.

Start by looking through your food cupboard and getting rid of unhealthy food: the high sugar and high saturated fat foods and replace these with fruit and vegetables. Fresh, frozen, and canned all are good so long as they are as natural as possible without additives or sugar. Buy as many different coloured vegetables and start eating high plant-based meals.

Replace high saturated fats with olive oil or other healthy oils and fats: including nuts and avocados. Eat lean organic meat, chicken, low-fat beef, lamb, and fresh fish.

Make healthy meals with these ingredients supplemented with wholemeal bread, brown rice, and brown pasta. As a result, you may lose weight and your skin will become clearer and healthier. Your whole sense of well-being will improve.

What follows from that? Exercise is pleasurable and your mind becomes clearer. As you exercise, solutions to your worries come into your head. You find answers to challenges that have been causing you stress and you know exactly what you will do.

Looking after your body affects your mind and that in turn improves your spiritual and emotional well-being too. You will notice and marvel at sunrises and sunsets and the changing seasons throughout the year.

All these wonderful benefits happen by changing your diet mindfully and knowing you are doing this because you want to live in a healthy body and look after your mind and spirit too. However, the unexpected outcome is that you eat what you need to become the weight you truly want to be.

Body, mind, or spirit? Which one holds the key to true fulfilment and happiness?

While each component plays a vital role in your overall well-being, the answer ultimately lies in finding a harmonious balance between all three.

Your body represents your physical health, fitness, and appearance. Taking care of your body through wholesome nutrition, regular exercise, and self-care practice is vital. A healthy body allows you to pursue your passions, and experience happiness through physical activities.

Simultaneously, your mind serves as your mental and intellectual sense. It includes your thoughts, emotions, beliefs, and ability to reason and process information. Nurturing your mind involves continuous learning, mental stimulation, emotional regulation, and experiencing meditation or mindfulness. A healthy mind enables you to cope with the difficulties of life, make sound decisions, and maintain a positive outlook.

Lastly, the spirit represents your inner essence, your connection to something greater than yourself. It encompasses your values, beliefs, passions, and sense of purpose. Cultivating your spirit involves introspection, self-reflection, exploring spiritual practices, and aligning with your core values. A healthy spirit provides you with a profound sense of meaning, fulfilment, and a feeling of interconnectedness with the universe.

True fulfilment and happiness arise when all three aspects are nourished and in harmony. Neglecting one component can lead to imbalance, leaving you feeling incomplete and discontented. For instance, if you focus solely on physical appearance at the expense of your mental and spiritual well-being, you may find yourself trapped in a cycle of shallow satisfaction and constant striving for external validation.

It is essential to recognise that fulfilment comes from within, and no single aspect can provide lasting happiness. By integrating physical health, mental well-being, and spiritual growth into your life, you create a full approach to self-care. This allows you to live realistically, with a sense of purpose, and achieve a higher level of contentment. Ultimately, the key to true fulfilment and happiness lies in recognising the interconnectedness of your body, mind, and spirit. By nurturing these aspects and finding a delicate balance, you can unlock your greatest potential and lead a fulfilling and meaningful life.

17. Hypnosis for weight loss.

———

Hypnosis is a useful tool to change habits that need a change of mindset for you to succeed.

During hypnosis relax each part of your body from your feet up through your legs, abdomen, arms, chest, shoulders, face, and head, as you are hypnotised.

During a hypnotic trance, the sub-conscious mind accepts suggestions so after hypnosis there is a greater ability to achieve. Hypnosis is useful for general stress management as well as weight loss. You will have suggestions made to you that, for example, certain foods, taste disgusting, or you will think of it wrapped in dust and imagine it full of maggots.

During hypnosis you will go into a state of deep relaxation but will be aware of everything said to you. You will not be asleep. When you come out of the trance state you will find your mindset will be different and it is easier to make the changes you want.

Hypnosis for weight loss is a natural and effective approach to achieving lasting weight loss. It taps into the power of your subconscious mind, creating lasting changes in your thoughts, behaviours, and beliefs related to food, exercise, and self-image. By using the power of your mind, you can overcome obstacles and achieve your weight loss goals with ease and confidence.

Through deep relaxation techniques, it will help you quiet your conscious mind and reach a state where your subconscious is open to suggestions. During this process, it will address any negative beliefs or thoughts about weight loss, replacing them with empowering affirmations and visualisation exercises that will support your progress.

Often, your relationship with food is emotional and deeply ingrained. Hypnosis helps you explore your triggers, desires, and patterns surrounding food and eliminate unhealthy cravings or emotional connections. Using visualisation and positive suggestions, it will reprogramme your subconscious mind to make healthier choices, appreciate nourishing foods, and feel satisfied with smaller portions.

Weight loss is not only about physical habits; it is also influenced by emotional well-being. With hypnosis, you will address any emotional blocks or traumas, such as stress, anxiety, or emotional eating, that may be hindering your progress. Through powerful hypnosis techniques, you will release negative emotions, replace them with feelings of self-love and confidence, and create a stronger foundation for your weight loss.

Building healthy habits and staying motivated are vital for long-term weight loss success. Hypnosis will enable you to programme your subconscious mind to embrace regular exercise, enjoy physical activities, and maintain an active lifestyle. By visualising your future self and setting clear goals, you will enhance your motivation, discipline, and determination to achieve your ideal weight and maintain it effortlessly.

A positive body image and self-esteem are essential for maintaining weight loss and a healthy lifestyle. You will work on strengthening your self-image, boosting self-confidence, and promoting a sense of body acceptance. By using visualisation techniques, you will develop a deep appreciation for your body, increase self-care, and radiate confidence from within.

Hypnosis enables you to take the first step towards transforming your relationship with food, body, and weight. With the power of hypnosis and your subconscious mind, you can make profound changes and achieve the weight loss you desire.

18. Can coaching help weight loss?

Would life coaching be useful to help you lose weight? You may wonder if there is an alternative to 'going on a diet' to reach the weight you want to be.

Instead of yet another diet, a coach could help you change your mindset about your weight.

Since being overweight is as much about balance, especially between the amount of exercise you do and the quantity and quality of your food, techniques which would help you have a better balance in your life are useful for weight loss.

Being overweight may be related to emotional eating. It would be logical to assume that better balance, less frustration and time to do more of what you want can all be useful to enable you to stop over-eating in response to emotional upset because you would not use food for comfort.

You could benefit from coaching around your life balance even if you are the sort of person who likes to sort things out for themselves without involving someone who doesn't know you.

Here are the questions to ask yourself to help you decide whether to try coaching.

What is the one change you can make? There is usually one thing which you know would make a huge difference not only about your weight but also your life.

What can you stop and what could you do less? If you ban something completely you are more likely to crave it.

What can you do today to make a difference? Having a walk for 15 minutes would be easy to do and have healthy effects.

Discover what's stopping you and remove those obstacles.

Are you frustrated with countless unsuccessful attempts at losing weight?

Do you find it difficult to stick to a diet or exercise routine?

If so, a weight loss coach may be just what you need to finally achieve your goals.

Coaching for weight loss helps you develop habits to enable you to reach your target weight.

A weight loss coach is someone who will guide and support you throughout your weight loss, providing valuable knowledge, accountability, and motivation.

A weight loss coach will work with you to create a tailored plan based on your unique needs, preferences, and lifestyle. They will assess your current habits, and help you identify potential barriers, and ways to overcome them. This ensures that the plan is realistic and achievable for you.

One of the main benefits of a weight loss coach is the built-in accountability. Your coach will regularly check in with you, track your progress, and help you stay on track. This level of accountability increases your chances of success and helps you stay motivated even when faced with challenges.

A weight loss coach is an expert in nutrition, exercise, and behaviour change. They will provide you with valuable information and educate you on the best practices for achieving weight loss. This knowledge empowers you to make informed decisions about your health and ensures that you are equipped with the right tools for long-term success.

Losing weight can be challenging and it's easy to get discouraged along the way. A weight loss coach is there to provide ongoing support and motivation. They will celebrate your successes, inspire you to keep going and help you overcome obstacles that arise.

Coaching for weight loss focuses on creating sustainable lifestyle changes. Instead of relying on fad diets or extreme exercise routines, a weight loss coach will help you build healthy habits that you can maintain for the long term. This approach not only helps you achieve your goal weight but also ensures that you maintain your progress and avoid the common cycle of weight regain.

If you're ready to make a lasting change in your life and achieve your weight loss goals, consider working with a weight loss coach. With their guidance, knowledge, and support, you'll have the tools you need to transform your lifestyle, improve your health, and finally attain the weight you desire.

19. Energy and motivation

———

To get all your tasks done and have the energy and motivation to do other things you want to achieve, you must have plenty of energy. You need enough energy to keep going for a huge number of hours every day so that you remain alert and efficient however many hours you've already been working.

What are the essentials for maintaining energy and being able to work efficiently yet still have a reserve of energy for your out-of-work activities?

In essence, the maintenance of energy boils down to the basics of looking after your mind, your body and spirit. Although this may be different for different people, it can be summarised as eating well, exercising regularly and relaxing.

This means eating healthy food regularly, and not poisoning your body with excess alcohol, and high-fat food with little nutritional value. it's important to keep your blood sugar at a good level by having something to eat every 2 to 3 hours. Your body, mind and spirit will not benefit from you working through the lunch hour forgetting to have breakfast.

Maintaining your energy levels will increase your efficiency because you will think more clearly and work more quickly.

Although you may get a certain amount of exercise when you walk around during the day, you need to ensure to take a walk every day.

As well as walking you may decide to go to a gym regularly or do some other form of exercise such as yoga. When you move your body, even if you are feeling tired, the outcome is very often a feeling of increased energy.

Practice relaxation, meditation, and connect with nature, to refresh your spirit.

By doing these things regularly you will have the energy to get more done during your day and to enjoy your life much more.

What small change do you need to introduce into your life, your week, or your day, to enhance your health and well-being?

Remember there may not be an instant result but drop by drop, bit by bit, small steps will contribute to the larger result. You must start somewhere, with something however small.

Energy and motivation are crucial factors in achieving weight loss. While changing your lifestyle and habits can be challenging, maintaining high energy levels, and staying motivated will help you stay on track and reach your weight loss goals.

Here are some tips to boost your energy and keep your motivation strong throughout achieving weight loss:

Break down your weight loss goals into smaller, achievable targets. It can be discouraging to set lofty goals that are difficult to attain. Start with small milestones and celebrate each success along the way.

Remind yourself of the reasons why you want to lose weight. Whether it's improving your health, boosting your self-confidence, or being able to keep up with your kids, having a clear WHY will give you purpose and help you stay motivated.

Surround yourself with positive and supportive people who can cheer you on and provide encouragement. Join weight loss groups or seek out friends or family members who have similar goals. Sharing your experiences with others can help you feel accountable and motivated.

Create a schedule for your meals and exercise routine. Planning helps eliminate decision fatigue and ensures you have the energy to make healthy choices. This also allows you to prioritise physical activity and make it a vital part of your day.

Dehydration can lead to fatigue and low energy levels. Make sure to drink enough water throughout the day to keep your body hydrated and your energy levels up. It is recommended to drink at least eight glasses of water daily.

Prioritise quality sleep to recharge and renew your energy levels. Lack of sleep can lead to increased cravings for unhealthy foods and lower motivation to engage in physical activities.

Celebrate your progress, no matter how small. Remember that weight loss is a process, and setbacks are a part of it. Focus on the positive changes you are making in your life, both physically and mentally.

Try new exercises or activities to keep your workouts exciting and prevent boredom. Include different exercises like strength training, cardio, and yoga to challenge your body and keep motivation high.

Treat yourself for reaching milestones or achieving specific goals. Rewarding yourself with non-food-related incentives, such as a massage or a new piece of clothing, will help you stay motivated and reinforce positive behaviours.

Create a mental image of how you want to look and feel at your goal weight. Visualising yourself achieving success can be a powerful motivator. Use visualisation techniques to imagine the positive changes you will experience and the benefits you will gain from reaching your weight loss goals.

Weight loss requires determination. By staying energised and motivated, you can overcome challenges and achieve the healthy, fit body you desire.

20. The mental energy to lose weight.

———

How can you gain the mental energy to lose weight?
To successfully lose weight, it's important to approach this with determination. Gaining the mental energy to lose weight can help you stay motivated, well-organised, and focused on your goals.

Here are a few strategies to help you boost your mental energy and lead the way for weight loss success:

Start by setting clear, achievable, and measurable goals that align with your long-term vision. Make sure your goals are meaningful to you and go beyond just the number on the scale. For example, focus on improving your overall health, increasing your energy levels, or enhancing your self-confidence.

Take the time to visualise yourself achieving your weight loss goals. Imagine how you will feel, the improved health benefits you'll experience, and the positive impact it will have on your life. Visualisation can boost your motivation and mental energy.

Surround yourself with positivity and eliminate your self-sabotaging thoughts. Practice positive affirmations, such as "I am capable of achieving my weight loss goals" or "I have the power to make healthy choices." Train your mind to focus on the positive aspects of your weight loss rather than dwelling on past failures or setbacks.

Educate yourself: Gain knowledge about nutrition, exercise, and healthy lifestyle habits. Understanding how your body works and how different food choices can impact your weight can be empowering.

Educating yourself will not only provide you with the necessary information but will also increase your confidence and motivation.

Build a support network: Share your weight loss experiences with a reliable support network. Surround yourself with people who motivate you. Having someone to encourage you, hold you accountable, and share your successes and challenges will help your mental energy and make your progress more enjoyable and long-lasting.

Prioritise self-care that helps you recharge and rejuvenate. Get enough sleep, engage in stress-reducing activities like yoga or meditation, indulge in hobbies you enjoy, and take breaks when needed. Taking care of your mental and emotional well-being will provide you with the mental energy necessary to stay committed to your weight loss goals.

Recognise and celebrate your achievements along the way, no matter how small. Acknowledge every positive change and milestone you reach. Celebrating these wins will boost your confidence, reinforce your progress, and increase your mental energy.

Gaining the mental energy to lose weight is a continuous process that requires patience, perseverance, and self-care. By implementing these strategies and staying committed, you can overcome any mental barriers and pave the way for weight loss success.

21. Your microbiome.

─────

Your gut microbiome is the trillions of microorganisms that reside in your digestive system. These tiny organisms play a crucial role in your overall health and well-being. To ensure a healthy gut microbiome, it's important to take proper care of it. Here are some tips for looking after your gut microbiome:

Eat a diverse range of foods: A balanced diet rich in a variety of fruits, vegetables, whole grains, and lean proteins will help support a diverse gut microbiome. Different types of fibre found in plant-based foods act as fuel for the beneficial bacteria in your gut, promoting their growth and diversity.

Include fermented foods: Foods like yoghurt, sauerkraut, kimchi, kefir, and miso are fermented and contain live bacteria that can positively influence your gut microbiome. Including these foods in your diet can help introduce beneficial bacteria into your gut and improve its overall health.

Avoid excessive use of antibiotics: Antibiotics are designed to kill harmful bacteria, but they can also negatively impact the beneficial bacteria in your gut. Whenever possible, try to avoid unnecessary antibiotic use or discuss alternative treatments with your healthcare professional.

Limit processed and sugary foods: These foods tend to be low in fibre and rich in additives, preservatives, and artificial sweeteners. Consuming excessive amounts of processed and sugary foods can negatively affect your gut microbiome, leading to an imbalance of bacteria.

Manage your stress levels: Stress can have a significant impact on your gut health. Chronic stress can disrupt the balance of bacteria in your gut, leading to various digestive issues. Engaging in stress-reducing activities like meditation, yoga, or regular exercise can help promote a healthier gut.

Stay hydrated: Drinking an adequate amount of water throughout the day is essential for optimal gut health. Water helps to flush out waste and supports proper digestion and nutrient absorption. Aim to drink at least eight glasses of water daily.

Poor sleep has been linked to an imbalance in gut bacteria. Aim for seven to nine hours of quality sleep each night to help maintain a healthy gut microbiome.

Regular physical activity not only benefits your overall health but also promotes a healthy gut microbiome. Exercise has been shown to increase the diversity of gut bacteria, contributing to improved gut health.

Remember, everyone's gut microbiome is unique, so it's important to listen to your body and adjust accordingly. If you're experiencing persistent digestive concerns, it's best to consult your doctor for advice and guidance. Taking care of your gut microbiome can support your overall health and well-being.

22. Avoid ultra-processed food

Avoiding ultra-processed food is crucial for maintaining a healthy diet and overall well-being. Ultra-processed foods are typically high in added sugars, unhealthy fats, and artificial additives while lacking essential nutrients. Here are some tips to help you avoid these types of food:

Read food labels: Ultra-processed foods often contain a long list of unrecognisable ingredients. Before purchasing any packaged food, check the ingredients list and avoid products that contain excessive amounts of added sugars, artificial sweeteners, preservatives, and unhealthy fats.

Opt for homemade meals using fresh ingredients whenever possible. Prepare your meals to have complete control over the ingredients used and ensure you're consuming real, whole foods.

Choose whole foods: Focus on consuming whole foods such as fruits, vegetables, whole grains, lean proteins, and healthy fats. These foods provide essential nutrients and are less likely to be processed or contain added sugars and unhealthy fats.

Avoid pre-packaged meals and snacks: Ready-made frozen meals, packaged snacks, and fast food tend to be highly processed. Limit your consumption of these convenient but unhealthy options and opt for homemade alternatives or healthier takeout options when needed.

Be alert to hidden sugars: Ultra-processed foods often contain high amounts of hidden sugars, such as in sodas, processed juices, flavoured yoghurts, and breakfast cereals. Read nutrition labels carefully and opt for products with no added sugars or those made from natural sweeteners, such as fruit or honey.

Be cautious of "low-fat" or "diet" products: Many low-fat or diet food products compensate for the reduction in fat by adding extra sugar, artificial sweeteners, or other additives. These can be just as harmful as the fat they aim to reduce. Instead, choose naturally low-fat foods or moderate portion sizes of healthier fats like avocados, nuts, and seeds.

Stay hydrated: Instead of reaching for sugary drinks or processed juices, hydrate yourself with plain water, herbal teas, or infused water with fresh fruit slices or herbs.

While it may be impossible to eliminate ultra-processed foods from your diet, making a conscious effort to minimise their consumption and focusing on whole, unprocessed foods can greatly improve your health and well-being.

23. Risk of relapse

———

Have you had the experience of being successful at losing weight while you were a member of a slimming club for a few months, only to regain all the weight lost when you stopped attending?

It seems like a plot to keep you paying to maintain your weight loss.

So, to retain your success, you need to do more than go to a slimming club or follow a weight loss diet.

It's about realising that diets on their own won't work in the long term. Yes, if you follow what is written, or what you're told, you will lose weight. However, in most cases, the weight is regained very quickly once you decide you're going back to a "normal" diet.

If diets don't work, then what can you do to be the weight you would like to be and healthy too?

The risk of relapse after losing weight is a common concern among individuals who have successfully shed unwanted pounds. While weight loss itself is an achievement, maintaining weight loss in the long term can prove to be challenging.

Several factors contribute to the risk of relapse after losing weight. Firstly, the body's natural defence mechanisms often work against weight loss, as they tend to promote weight regain. These mechanisms include hormonal changes that increase appetite and promote fat storage, making it harder to sustain the weight loss achieved. Additionally, the body's metabolism can slow down after weight loss, making it easier to regain weight.

Another factor that increases the risk of relapse is the psychological aspect of losing weight. Many individuals experience a sense of achievement and euphoria after successfully losing weight, which can lead to complacency or a relaxed attitude towards their weight maintenance efforts. This may result in returning to old habits, such as unhealthy eating patterns or a sedentary lifestyle.

External factors can also contribute to the risk of relapse. Social and environmental influences, such as the availability of high-calorie foods and a lack of support from friends and family, can make it more challenging to maintain a healthy lifestyle after weight loss. Additionally, stress, emotional eating, and lack of time for self-care can all increase the likelihood of relapse.

To lessen the risk of relapse, it is crucial to adopt workable lifestyle changes rather than relying on fad diets. This involves making long-term changes to eating habits, incorporating regular physical activity, and finding healthier ways to cope with stress and emotions. It is also essential to establish a strong support system, whether it be through friends, family, or professional guidance.

Monitoring progress and maintaining accountability can be helpful as well. Keeping track of eating habits, exercise routines, and weight fluctuations allows for early detection of any potential setback and provides an opportunity to adjust before significant weight regain occurs.

The chance of relapse after losing weight is a valid concern. However, if you focus on positive lifestyle changes, you can reduce the risk and maintain your weight loss successfully.

24. Reasons to stop dieting.

———

Here are some reasons why diets don't work:
Diets don't work in the long term: you may lose some weight while you are on the diet, but it goes back on plus more when you come off the diet.

You can't restrict certain foods forever: you need to eat food from each group: carbohydrates, fats, and protein, so a diet restricting any of these will lead to cravings and overeating.

Counting calories or points is OK when you are at home but virtually impossible when you are eating in a restaurant, so you may be wrongly estimating how much you are consuming.

By forbidding certain foods you may develop such a strong desire to eat them that you end up eating far too much.

Diets are often unsustainable in the long term. Many require restrictive eating patterns or the elimination of certain food groups, which can lead to feelings of deprivation and eventually result in binge eating or falling back into old eating habits.

Constantly focusing on restriction and counting calories can create an unhealthy obsession with food and lead to guilt and shame when straying from the diet plan.

Diets can negatively impact mental health. The stress and pressure of sticking to a strict diet can contribute to increased anxiety and even lead to the development of disordered eating patterns or eating disorders.

Diets often ignore individual needs. Each person's body is unique and has different nutritional requirements. Following a one-size-fits-all diet may not address specific dietary needs or health conditions, potentially leading to nutritional deficiencies or worsening of existing health issues.

Diets often result in weight cycling or "yo-yo dieting." Weight loss and regain cycles can be harmful to physical health and ultimately make it harder to maintain a healthy weight in the long run.

Diets do not address the root cause of unhealthy eating habits. Dieting focuses on the external solution of weight loss, but it often fails to address the emotional and psychological reasons behind overeating or unhealthy food choices. Without addressing these underlying issues, long-term success is unlikely.

Diets can lead to a preoccupation with body image. The constant emphasis on achieving a certain body shape or size can add to body dissatisfaction and contribute to low self-esteem.

Diets can affect metabolism. Rapid weight loss from severe calorie restriction can slow down the metabolism, making it harder to lose weight in the future and increasing the chances of weight regain.

Diets overlook the importance of overall well-being. True health goes beyond just weight loss. It includes mental and emotional well-being, physical fitness, and enjoying a balanced and varied diet. Focusing solely on weight loss often neglects these other essential aspects of a healthy lifestyle.

Instead of dieting, adopting a balanced and sustainable approach to eating is more beneficial in the long run. Listening to your body's hunger and fullness cues, practising mindful eating, and making informed food choices can all contribute to a healthier relationship with food and long-term well-being.

25. Alternatives to dieting.

———

Here are some no-diet ways to lose weight:

- Eat only when you are genuinely hungry.
- What do you need when you reach for food?
- Are you thirsty rather than hungry?
- Drink more water.
- Distinguish food hunger and emotional hunger.
- Deal with emotional hunger.

- Enjoy what you eat.
- Say no when you don't want to eat.
- Eat mindfully.

Intuitive eating: This approach focuses on listening to your body's natural hunger and fullness cues, rather than following strict diet rules. You eat when you're hungry and stop when you're satisfied, while also allowing yourself to enjoy all types of foods in moderation.

Mindful eating involves paying full attention to the eating experience. It involves eating slowly, savouring each bite, and being fully present in the moment. By practicing mindful eating, you can develop a healthier relationship with food and be more in tune with your body's needs.

Aim for well-rounded and balanced food. Consume a variety of nutrient-dense foods, including fruits, vegetables, whole grains, lean proteins, and healthy fats, to ensure you're getting all the necessary nutrients your body needs.

Rather than eliminating foods or counting calories, focus on portion sizes. Use smaller plates and bowls to visually trick your brain into thinking you're eating more.

Pay attention to your body's fullness cues and stop eating once you're satisfied, rather than clearing your plate.

Incorporate regular physical activity to promote overall health and maintain a healthy weight. Engage in activities you enjoy, such as walking, swimming, dancing, or playing a sport, to make exercise a sustainable and enjoyable part of your lifestyle.

Focus on adopting healthy habits rather than fixating on weight loss. This can include drinking plenty of water, getting enough sleep, managing stress, and avoiding excessive alcohol or sugar consumption. By prioritising overall wellness, weight management can become a natural by-product.

Seek support and accountability by joining communities focused on overall health and well-being. Sharing your experiences, challenges, and successes with like-minded individuals provides motivation and guidance on your way towards a healthier lifestyle.

26. New Year resolutions.

———

D o you decide each year that this will be the year that you'll reach a healthy weight and keep it off?

What happens after the initial enthusiasm and how can you keep motivated to achieve your goal and keep to a healthy weight?

Instead of your goals being around the weight you want to be, set them about changing your habits and beliefs about weight.

Introduce a positive change. Build on your new healthy eating habits each week. Don't change everything at once. Remember it can take at least twenty-one days for a new habit to embed itself into your unconscious mind.

Increase the amount of exercise you do. Make it simple such as parking further away from the shops, getting off the bus sooner than you need to and taking a walk around the block each day.

Notice your self-talk. What do you say to yourself? Make sure you make positive statements such as 'I am confident.' 'I am gaining a healthy weight', rather than 'Losing weight is difficult' or I'm going to fail again.'

Remember to have a life. Get your mind in the right frame by really enjoying the taste of healthy food so that eating more healthily is a pleasure not a chore.

Clear your clothes cupboard of what you no longer need. This includes large clothes which no longer fit and small clothes you may never wear again. Both will delay your weight loss efforts: the large clothes because keeping these reinforces the message that you will relapse, put on weight again and go back to wearing them. The small clothes may represent an unobtainable goal if they date back many years previously when you were much younger and had a very differently shaped body. Instead, as you achieve the weight you desire, treat yourself to one or two new items of clothing.

Get rid of mental clutter. Change the conversation with yourself, negative messages about never being able to lose weight clutter your mind. Replace them with affirmations such as 'every day I become fitter and healthier'.

Instead of aiming for drastic weight loss, set a realistic goal of losing 1-2 pounds per week. This slow and steady approach is more sustainable and healthier in the long run.

Focus on incorporating a variety of fruits, vegetables, lean proteins, whole grains, and healthy fats into your meals. Aim for portion control and avoid sugary and ultra-processed foods.

Drinking enough water throughout the day helps boost metabolism, curb appetite, and keep you feeling fuller for longer. Aim for at least 8 glasses of water per day.

Incorporate physical activity into your daily routine. Aim for at least 150 minutes of moderate-intensity exercise per week, such as brisk walking, cycling, or swimming. Additionally, include strength training exercises to build muscle mass and increase metabolism.

Getting sufficient sleep is important for weight loss and overall health. Aim for 7-9 hours of quality sleep each night to avoid fatigue and cravings for unhealthy foods.

Keep track of your progress. Documenting your meals, exercise routine, and weight fluctuations can help you stay accountable and identify patterns that may affect weight loss. Consider using a food diary or a smartphone app to track your progress.

Think about joining a weight loss support group, partnering with a workout buddy, or seeking the guidance of a registered dietitian or personal trainer. Having support can help keep you motivated and focused on your goal.

Practice mindful eating by slowing down during meals, savouring each bite, and listening to your body's hunger and fullness cues. Avoid mindless eating in front of screens or eating out of emotional triggers.

Find healthy alternatives: Instead of reaching for sugary snacks or processed foods, find healthier alternatives. For example, replace sugary drinks with herbal teas or fruit-infused water, or swap chips for air-popped popcorn.

Be consistent and patient: Remember that losing weight takes time and effort. Stay consistent with your healthy habits, even if progress is slow. Celebrate small victories along the way and don't get discouraged by setbacks. Patience and persistence are key to reaching your weight loss goals.

27. A new way of eating.

I f you are aiming to introduce a new way of eating into your life, be realistic: it may take a month or more before you do it automatically.

Do you remember learning to drive a car? How at first you went through all the procedures very deliberately, until eventually after some time, you drive almost automatically. You may not even realise how you got to your destination because you are on 'automatic pilot'.

Don't give up too soon on the new eating habits that will improve your life by enabling you to lose the weight you've been struggling with for years. Use a chart to tick off the days and you will find that after twenty to thirty days you are repeating the new habit without even thinking about it.

When you decide on introducing a new habit don't forget SMART goals. Be SPECIFIC about what you want. Make the attainment of your goal MEASURABLE, ACHIEVABLE and REALISTIC for you to reach in a certain TIME. If, for example, your goal is to eat breakfast every day then make that goal more specific by saying exactly what you will eat. You could say a bowl of cereal plus a piece of fruit depending on what you have available. You can measure your success by noting each day as you succeed in what you set out to do.

By being specific you will be able to make sure you have bought the necessary supplies so you can have those available for breakfast each day.

For every goal during your weight loss, there is more than just deciding not to follow a strict diet anymore. Since you will be eating more healthily plan what to buy so that there isn't the temptation to eat unsuitable foods. Say no to 'diet' and 'yes' to changing your eating habits one step at a time.

Take the time to plan your meals ahead of time. Consider the ingredients, flavours, and nutritional value of each meal. This helps you make informed choices and ensures a balanced diet.

Instead of focusing on the quantity of food you consume, prioritise the quality of ingredients. Choose whole, unprocessed foods. This not only improves your overall health but also amplifies the enjoyment of your meals.

Eating mindfully involves slowing down, chewing thoroughly, and paying attention to the sensations in your mouth. Take the time to appreciate the textures, flavours, and aromas of each bite. This practice enhances your eating experience and allows you to feel more satisfied with less food.

Incorporate foods that bring you joy and pleasure. Whether it's a square of dark chocolate, a serving of your favourite comfort food, or a delicious homemade dessert, allowing yourself to indulge in moderation is an essential part of this approach.

Listen to your body. Eat when you're hungry and stop when you're comfortably full. This eliminates the need for strict portion control or calorie counting, promoting a healthier and more balanced relationship with food.

Snacking mindfully is just as important as mindful eating at meals. Choose nutritious snacks that satisfy your cravings and provide nourishment. Take the time to enjoy them fully, free from distractions, and be aware of portion sizes.

Eating is often a communal experience meant to be shared with others. Connect with loved ones over meals, developing a sense of community and joy around food.

Transform your eating habits into a pleasurable experience. No more restrictive diets or guilt-ridden meals. It's time to savour every bite, nourish your body, and create a positive relationship with food that lasts a lifetime.

28. What does success mean to you?

———

W hether your idea of success is related to losing weight or living the life you truly want, it's important to clarify what you want in life.

Success, no matter what it may mean to you, can result in more happiness and more emotional fulfilment. It may lead to more financial and non-financial rewards too.

Remember that success means different things to people, so it's important to clarify what it means to you. It's your life so don't fall into the trap of aiming for someone else's definition of success. Your ideas about what success means can change as you reach different stages in your life.

One of the most important things you need to engage with is what you think about yourself now, and the difference you expect when you achieve the healthy weight you're aiming for.

Success and confidence won't magically appear after you've lost weight. Do what you can now to feel better about yourself and to increase your self-confidence.

Imagine yourself in the future, if you do nothing about your weight, and look back at yourself in the present time. What advice would the future you give to the present you?

You may have consulted an 'ideal weight' chart and realise that there is little chance you will achieve that weight. Success may be defined instead by being able to wear a particular item of clothing rather than a precise number on the weighing scales.

- Define what success means to you.
- List several ways to succeed.
- Choose the way which appeals most to you.
- What is stopping you from achieving?
- What will you do to remove the obstacles?
- When will you take the first step?
- When do you plan to achieve your goal?

By doing this you will have a strategy for change and a plan to follow. This technique will be even more successful if you write down the stages defined above and note your progress each day.

29. Change your mind and your weight.

———

Weight loss is a common goal for many people. Achieving and maintaining it can be challenging.

Instead of focusing on diets and exercise routines, don't overlook the importance of the mind-body connection. Shifting your mindset plays a crucial role in changing your weight. Doing this can positively impact your relationship with food, exercise, and overall well-being.

Changing your mind to change your weight shifts your perspective on weight loss. Instead of viewing it as a temporary fix or a quick solution, you understand that it is long-term. By adopting a positive mindset and acknowledging that weight loss is an all-inclusive process, you can set realistic goals and make sustainable changes.

Self-acceptance is vital when it comes to changing your weight. While attempting this, it is essential to appreciate and respect your body as it is. Developing a positive self-image allows you to make healthier choices motivated by self-care, not self-criticism.

Negative thoughts can hinder your progress and motivation in weight loss. Identify and challenge the negative beliefs surrounding food, exercise, and body image. Instead of focusing on limitations, focus on the possibilities and the transformation ahead.

Mindful eating involves bringing awareness to your eating habits, food choices, and how full you feel. Slow down, savour each bite, and listen to your body's signals of hunger and fullness. By becoming more attuned to your body's needs, you can develop a healthier relationship with food and make conscious choices that align with your weight goals.

Exercise should be seen as an enjoyable activity rather than a chore. Find physical activities that you genuinely enjoy, whether it's dancing, swimming, hiking, or yoga. By shifting your mindset to view exercise as an opportunity for personal growth and self-expression, you are more likely to stick to it and reap the benefits of an active lifestyle.

Surround yourself with positive and supportive people. Seek out like-minded individuals who share similar goals or find a mentor who can guide you through your weight loss experiences. Sharing your successes, challenges, and experiences with others can provide encouragement, accountability, and the motivation you need to stay on track.

Changing your mind is the key to changing your weight sustainably. By adopting a positive mindset, practising self-acceptance, challenging negative thoughts, cultivating mindful eating habits, finding joy in exercise, and seeking support, you can transform your relationship with weight loss.

It's not just about shedding pounds; it's about developing a positive and lasting change in your overall well-being. With the right frame of mind, accept that change is possible and that you can do what you need to do.

Don't miss out!

Visit the website below and you can sign up to receive emails whenever Susan Kersley publishes a new book. There's no charge and no obligation.

https://books2read.com/r/B-A-EFNC-CDWWC

BOOKS 2 READ

Connecting independent readers to independent writers.

Did you love *Mind Over Weight*? Then you should read *Improve Your Work Life Balance*[1] by Susan Kersley!

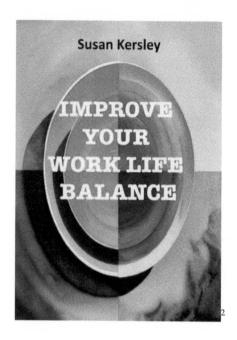

[2]

Many people feel unhappy about the state of their work-life balance. Perhaps you're one of them, and like them, you may want to know what you could do to restore, rebuild, and renew it.

If your work is your life and you have no time for little else, then something must change. Work is important and may take up many waking hours. But don't neglect the rest. It is vital to find time for your friends and family, your partner, and your community. But most important of all is you and what is essential for your health and happiness.

---

1. https://books2read.com/u/mBAqzZ

2. https://books2read.com/u/mBAqzZ

That means discovering the steps you need to take to make a difference. It entails making time for parts of your life that you ignore. It involves committing yourself to making changes.

Many people feel unhappy about the state of their work-life balance. Perhaps you're one of them, and like them, you may want to know what you could do to restore, rebuild, and renew it.

If your work is your life and you have no time for little else, then something must change. Work is important and may take up many waking hours. But don't neglect the rest. It is vital to find time for your friends and family, your partner, and your community. But most important of all is you and what is essential for your health and happiness.

That means discovering the steps you need to take to make a difference. It entails making time for parts of your life that you ignore. It involves committing yourself to making changes.

Many people feel unhappy about the state of their work-life balance. Perhaps you're one of them, and like them, you may want to know what you could do to restore, rebuild, and renew it.

If your work is your life and you have no time for little else, then something must change. Work is important and may take up many waking hours. But don't neglect the rest. It is vital to find time for your friends and family, your partner, and your community. But most important of all is you and what is essential for your health and happiness.

That means discovering the steps you need to take to make a difference. It entails making time for parts of your life that you ignore. It involves committing yourself to making changes.

Many people feel unhappy about the state of their work-life balance. Perhaps you're one of them, and like them, you may want to know what you could do to restore, rebuild, and renew it.

If your work is your life and you have no time for little else, then something must change. Work is important and may take up many waking hours. But don't neglect the rest. It is vital to find time for your friends and family, your partner, and your community. But most important of all is you and what is essential for your health and happiness.

That means discovering the steps you need to take to make a difference. It entails making time for parts of your life that you ignore. It involves committing yourself to making changes.

Read more at https://susankersley.co.uk.

Also by Susan Kersley

A Novel
Pills and Pillboxes
Connection Deception

Books about Weight Management
Weight Loss Success
Mind Over Weight

Books for Doctors
ABC of Change for Doctors
Life After Medicine
Prescription for Change
Work-Life Balance for Doctors
Lifestyle Coaching for Doctors
Meet the Challenges of Working as a Doctor
The Busy Doctor's Guide: Improve your Work-Life Balance

Retirement Books

Get Ready for Retirement
Life After Work
Retirement: Back to Basics

Self-help Books
How to Have a Balanced Life
69 Easy Ways to Change Your life
15 Ways to Change Your Life
Connect and Change
Coping With New Year Resolutions
More Time for You Now
How to Change Your Life
Improve Your Work Life Balance

Watch for more at https://susankersley.co.uk.

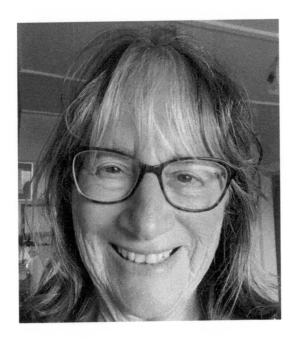

About the Author

Susan Kersley has written personal development and self-help books for doctors and others, and books about retirement and novels.

She was a doctor for thirty years and then left Medicine to be a Life Coach..

Now retired, she is updating her books and writing more. Please visit her website https://susankersley.co.uk

If you enjoyed this book, **please take a moment to leave a review.** Reviews are so important for independent authors.

Read more at https://susankersley.co.uk.

Milton Keynes UK
Ingram Content Group UK Ltd.
UKHW012016290224
438689UK00001B/82